I0846459

Yoga Studio Sensation
Opening and Operating a Successful Yoga Business

Table of Contents

Chapter 1. Introduction

Unleash your inner entrepreneur and channel your spirituality with our Special Report - "Yoga Studio Sensation: Opening and Operating a Successful Yoga Business". This joyful and enlightening guide is chock-full of insights and advice tailored to help you transform your dream into a reality. From envisioning your first yoga studio to managing the dynamics of the yoga business, we bring you a comprehensive roadmap to success. Peppered with real-life anecdotes and expert tips, this report is your handshake with prosperity and tranquility. Get ready to embark on a rewarding journey that harmonizes the body, mind, and wallet. Let's master your "Yoga-preneurship" one peaceful inhale and successful exhale at a time!

Chapter 2. Unlocking the Fundamentals of Yoga

In the journey towards becoming a successful Yoga-preneur, you must first understand the bedrock principles of yoga. Understanding the underlying fundamentals not only amplifies your knowledge but also empowers you to establish an authentic and meaningful yoga business.

2.1. The Origins of Yoga

Yoga, a Sanskrit word meaning 'union', arose over 5,000 years ago in Indus Valley Civilization. Rooted deeply in spirituality and philosophy, this practice was initially a method for spiritual growth and self-realization. Modern iterations have incorporated physical exercise, but the true essence of yoga lies beyond mere physicality. The primary texts associated with yoga include the Vedas, the Upanishads, The Bhagavad Gita, and the Yoga Sutras of Patanjali.

2.2. Yoga's Philosophical Foundations

Yoga revolves around holistic growth, encompassing spiritual, mental, and physical aspects. This philosophy is encapsulated in the Eight Limbs of Yoga clarified in Patanjali's Yoga Sutras:

1. Yama: Ethical standards or moral disciplines.

2. Niyama: Self-discipline and spiritual observance.

3. Asana: Posture or position designed to nurture the body.

4. Pranayama: Breathing exercises, energy control.

5. Pratyahara: Sensory withdrawal.

6. Dharana: Concentration.

7. Dhyana: Meditation or contemplation.

8. Samadhi: A state of ecstasy, a culmination of the previous seven practices.

Each limb is integral to the yoga practice and inspires a distinct essence of yoga which must be embraced as you build your yoga business.

2.3. Understanding Different Styles of Yoga

Different styles of yoga have been developed over time, each with unique characteristics:

1. Hatha Yoga: This is a classic approach to breathing and exercises. If a style of yoga is described as Hatha style, it likely focuses on the physical postures and breathing.

2. Vinyasa Yoga: Characterized by fluid transitions between postures, synchronized with the breath.

3. Yin Yoga: A slow-paced style, where poses are held for longer durations, aiming to work deeper into the muscles and connective tissues.

4. Ashtanga Yoga: A rigorous style following a specific sequence of postures.

5. Kundalini Yoga: A meditative style aiming to release the dormant energy within.

6. Restorative Yoga: A relaxing style focusing on body relaxation and healing.

Your yoga studio could focus on one or more styles, depending upon the clientele's preferences and your expertise.

2.4. Physical Aspects of Yoga: Asana and Pranayama

Asana, the practice of physical poses, is the most well-known aspect of yoga. Asanas range from gentler poses that aid relaxation and flexibility, to challenging poses that build strength and endurance. A firm understanding of asanas, their benefits, and the correct techniques are essential for a yoga studio owner.

Closely related to Asana is Pranayama, the practice of controlling the breath. Pranayama exercises are key to energizing, relaxing, and healing the mind and body. Being adept in pranayama techniques enhances your yoga teaching skills.

2.5. Mental Aspects of Yoga: Dharana and Dhyana

At its core, yoga is a tool to reach higher levels of consciousness and mental clarity. Dharana, the practice of concentration, and Dhyana, the practice of meditation, are significant to perform mindful yoga. By instilling them in your lessons, you provide your clients with tools to manage stress, increase self-awareness, and nurture peace within.

2.6. Conducting Yoga Sessions

Successful yoga sessions are those that do justice to the principles of yoga while catering to the needs of the practitioners. Sessions should be a balanced mix of asanas, pranayama, and meditation. Guiding your clients through the subtle nuances of body alignment, breath, and concentration makes the experience rewarding.

2.7. Vitality of Yoga Atmosphere and Environment

Creating the right environment for yoga practice is key – a clean, well-lit, and peaceful space. Incorporating elements like soft music, essential oils, yoga props can enhance the yoga experience.

With a firm grasp of the fundamentals, you would not just be opening a yoga studio. Instead, you would be creating a haven for those seeking physical well-being and mental tranquility. With each succeeding chapter, our guide will delve deeper into discovering the ins and outs of running a successful yoga studio. Let's yogify the world, one studio at a time!

Chapter 3. Conceptualizing Your Dream Yoga Studio

Behind every successful yoga studio, there is an initial dream. The conceptualization of this dream requires deep introspection, market research, and methodical planning. Rather than jump head-first into the world of "Yoga-preneurship", it is essential to lay sturdy groundwork that prospers your yoga business. This involves crafting your unique vision, understanding your audience, picking the right location, and identifying your resources. Let's dive in!

3.1. Crafting Your Unique Vision

A concrete and clear vision serves as a cornerstone in the creation of your dream yoga studio. Your vision will guide your decisions and actions, and provide inspiration.

But, how do you uncover this vision? Start with clarity over your own yoga journey. Dig deep and ask yourself about what yoga means to you, how it shapes your life, and how it can transform others' lives. Keep a note of the elements of yoga that resonate with you the most. This personal essence will differentiate your studio and make it special.

Beyond the personal realm, consider the broader impact. How will your studio serve the community? Will it target specific groups (seniors, kids, athletes)? Will you incorporate unique styles, like aerial yoga or yoga therapy? It is fundamental to align your personal and business vision. Draft a vision statement that imbues this ethos.

3.2. Understanding Your Audience

A clear understanding of your target audience enables the delivery of an attractive proposition. Your audience's demographics, interests, pain points, and yoga proficiency levels are pivotal.

Start exploring who your potential customers might be. Conduct demographic research on your local community. Use local statistics, social media insights, and market research reports. From age and gender to income ranges and lifestyle preferences - this knowledge is invaluable.

Next, examine their yoga levels. Are they beginners, intermediates, or advanced yogis? This sheds light on class levels and types. Touch base with potential customers through surveys or face-to-face interaction where possible. Unearth their motivations and challenges. What gives them peace and joy? What health problems they're struggling with? Answers to these stem your unique offerings.

3.3. Choosing the Right Location

Selecting the right location poses a significant impact on your yoga studio's visibility and accessibility. An incorrect choice can hamper your business growth.

A prime location caters to the convenience of your clientele. Research localities where your potential customers live or work. Also consider nearby amenities such as cafés or parks. Think about accessibility - is it connected through public transportation? These factors not only improve visibility but also foster a community-centric environment.

Do not neglect the ambiance. Flowing energy, tranquility, and space for your offerings are crucial. Remember, your studio will be a sanctuary for many. Select properties that align with your vision and can be adjusted to suit your potential themes and decor.

Also, take into account budget and local zoning laws. Hiring a professional real estate agent can aid in finding an optimal location within your budget.

3.4. Identifying Your Resources

Creating a yoga studio involves investment. Understanding your financial resources and developing a budget is a wise step. How much capital you need? What are your prospective revenue streams? What pricing models you will follow?

Include costs like property lease, renovations, licensing and permits, marketing and advertising, yoga gear, utilities, salaries, and insurance. Consider maintenance costs and potential unexpected expenses.

Ascertain your financing options. Bootstrapping, loans, crowdfunding, or partnerships? Ploughing back your earnings or external investments? These decisions aid in maintaining your studio's financial health.

In resources, consider other assets. Partnerships with local businesses or experienced yoga trainers? These partnerships can both reduce costs and add value.

Conceptualizing your yoga studio involves an intricate blend of your personal vision, market understanding, location tactics, and resource configuration. This chapter directs your contemplation in the initial step towards transforming your dream studio into a tangible reality. Stay tuned for the journey as we explore other chapters in creating an enrichable and profitable yoga business. Let's take our inhale as a symbol of invited challenges and exhale as a strong commitment to overcome them.

Chapter 4. Strategic Business Planning and Legalities

Understanding the importance of strategic planning and staying within legal boundaries are crucial for any business. The yoga studio business is no exception. In this journey towards becoming a Yoga-preneur, these aspects should be considered with utmost priority. Let's dive into this ocean of planning and legalities to ensure a safe sail towards your dream Yoga business.

4.1. Understanding Strategic Business Planning

Strategic business planning is the blueprint of your business. It paints a clear picture of what your business looks like currently, the goals you aim to achieve, and the steps you need to take to achieve them. It is a comprehensive long-term plan, bringing together the elements of feasibility, branding, marketing, finance, operational aspects and more into one detailed document.

1. **The Vision and Mission**: Begin this journey by defining what you foresee for your yoga studio. Understand your yoga philosophy, what you want to deliver through your yoga service and what your business stands for.

2. **Feasibility Analysis**: Evaluate the feasibility of your yoga studio. Look at factors such as the potential customer base, geographic location, and competition. You may want to conduct a SWOT analysis (Strengths, Weaknesses, Opportunities, Threats) to gain a well-rounded perspective.

3. **The Yoga Services**: Identify what type of yoga services will be offered. Are you focusing solely on yoga classes, or will you also provide yoga teacher training, workshops, and retreats?

4.2. Developing a Business Model

After defining the vision, it is important to build a sturdy business model canvas. This model should include your unique value proposition, customer segments, customer relationships, channels of delivery, cost structure, revenue streams, key partners, key activities, and key resources.

1. **Unique Value Proposition**: Your unique value proposition should define what sets you apart from other yoga studios.

2. **Revenue streams**: Understand where your income will come from. Will it be primarily from classes, memberships, workshops, or retail?

3. **Cost Structure**: Calculate your fixed and variable costs, including rent, utilities, salaries, and equipment.

4. **Channels of Delivery**: Identify how your services will reach customers. This could include in-studio classes, online platforms, or community programs.

4.3. Devising a Marketing & Sales Plan

Marketing and sales plans greatly influence your yoga studio's reach and revenues. Understand your target market, how you will reach them, the sales strategies you will adopt, and the revenue goals you have in place.

1. **Defining Target Market**: Develop a clear comprehension of who your clients will be. Based on this understanding, you can formulate engaging marketing strategies.

2. **Online Presence**: In this digital age, online presence is essential. This may involve investing in a professional website, selective digital advertising, and a strong social media presence.

3. **Revenue Goals**: Outline what your revenue targets are for the first year. This may vary by month, reflecting factors such as seasonal fluctuations.

4.4. Establishing Operational Procedures

The operational procedures should outline the daily operations of the business. This encompasses recruitment and training strategies, setting schedules, and maintenance of facilities.

4.5. Understanding Legalities

While dreaming big is important, it's equally essential to keep your business within the legal boundaries. Various aspects like registering your business, getting the required permits and licenses, obtaining the necessary insurance, understanding tax obligations, and protecting your intellectual property all fall under this crucial step.

1. **Registrations, Permits, and Licenses**: Ensure your yoga studio is legally equipped to deliver services. This could start from registering your yoga studio as a business entity to obtaining permits and licenses.

2. **Insurance**: Having a comprehensive insurance cover is vital for a yoga studio to safeguard your business from potential liabilities.

3. **Tax Obligations**: Understand what your tax obligations are, including income tax, Goods and Services Tax (GST), and levies.

4.6. Protecting Intellectual Property

While this may not immediately seem important to a yoga studio business, it can be a game-changer in the long run. Trademarks, copyrights, and patents can protect your unique practices, your branding, and your competitive difference.

By strategically planning and understanding the legalities, your dreams of running a successful yoga studio can transform into reality. This process ensures your vision is executable, financially viable, and legally sound. In the upcoming chapter, we will break down the financial planning and investment aspect for your future yoga business.

Chapter 5. Financial Foundations: Budgeting and Funding

Budgeting and funding are the bedrock of any business. Setting solid financial foundations is a matter of not just organising your resources but also of understanding how to put things into perspective. Before jumping into the world of yoga-preneurship, having a detailed plan for your budget and methods to acquire funding will ensure your business starts off with a strong financial footing and is prepared for future challenges.

5.1. Understanding the Costs

The first step in budgeting is understanding the kind of expenses you're likely to incur. This generally includes initial setup costs, rent or lease fees, equipment costs, costs for hiring and maintaining staff, marketing costs, insurance, and miscellaneous costs.

1. Initial setup costs: These include legal fees, licenses, permits, and the cost of renovating or decorating your yoga studio.

2. Rent or lease fees: The location of your studio greatly influences these costs. High-traffic, convenient locations tend to have high rent. If you're leasing the property, maintenance costs should also be considered.

3. Equipment costs: Mats, props, sound system, cleaning equipment, and software for scheduling and tracking customers will be some of your initial investments.

4. Hiring and maintaining staff: This includes salaries, benefits, and professional development or training costs.

5. Marketing costs: Brochures, posters, online ads, social media

promotions, and website maintenance fall under this category.

6. Insurance: It's crucial to have insurance cover to protect against possible damage or lawsuits.

7. Miscellaneous costs: These include utility costs (like heating for hot yoga classes), reception area costs, locker and relaxation area costs, and ongoing cleaning and maintenance.

Get quotes for these expenditures from various sources and consolidate them into a budget spreadsheet. This would give you a ballpark estimate of your initial and recurring costs.

5.2. Sourcing Funds

Think about where your funding is going to come from. There are several possible sources: personal funds, bank loans, investors, and crowdfunding. Be aware of the implications and obligations that each source carries.

1. Personal funds: These can come from savings or from liquidating assets. While the most straightforward source, it is also risky as it involves personal financial risk.

2. Bank loans: Traditional bank loans require a good credit history and collateral but offer lower interest rates. Alternatively, Small Business Administration loans offer various loan programs for start-ups.

3. Investors: This could be family, friends, or professional investors. They might offer funds in exchange for equity in your yoga business. It provides the capital with limited personal financial risk, but you'll have to relinquish some control over your business.

4. Crowdfunding: Platforms like Kickstarter and Indiegogo are modern ways to raise capital by appealing to a 'crowd' of people for small investments. You often provide some reward in return,

like free yoga classes.

5.3. Drafting a Budget

Once you understand your costs and potential sources of funding, draw up a detailed budget. Begin with one-time start-up costs followed by monthly recurring costs. This will help you assess the total initial investment needed and the ongoing monthly expenses to keep the yoga studio operational.

Don't forget to account for uncertainties and additional financial buffers. A helpful rule of thumb is to have a cash reserve to cover three to six months of expenses. This could help your business weather unforeseen circumstances or unexpected costs.

5.4. Business Plan

Your budget should be an integral part of your business plan. Illuminate the full financial picture of your yoga studio business to potential investors, lenders, or partners, and clearly communicate your strategic path to profitability.

5.5. Keeping Track of Your Finances

Once your yoga studio starts operations, track your finances meticulously. Compare actual costs against budgeted ones to identify cost overruns promptly. Use accounting software to save time and automate tasks. Keep a clear record of all transactions and review your bank statements regularly.

5.6. Exploring Partnership & Collaborations

Consider partnering with established wellness centers, corporate organizations, or schools to increase revenue. They could be interested in offering yoga classes for their members or employees as a wellness initiative.

5.7. Financial Review & Assessment

Regularly conduct a financial review to assess business performance and adjust strategies as necessary. This includes revisiting the budget, repayment plan, revenue growth, and cash flow management.

Remember, budgeting and funding your yoga studio is not a one-time event but a consistent practice that ensures long-term financial health. Considering the financial aspect comprehensively is like doing a balancing yoga pose - it brings awareness, focus, and ensures the stability of your yoga business.

Chapter 6. Location, Layout and Design: Making the Space Your Own

Transforming a simple space into a sanctuary dedicated to tranquility and internal growth is a crucial step in your yoga-preneurship journey. It's not just about choosing a location but creating an environment that resonates with peace, positivity, and purpose. Whether it's a vacant warehouse, a minimalistic loft, or a cozy corner in your home, your unique touch can transform it into a thriving yoga studio.

6.1. Choosing Your Location

When it comes to selecting a location for your yoga studio, consider three fundamental factors: Accessibility, Visibility, and Community. An ideal location is easily reachable, visible to potential customers, and embedded in a community that values wellness and fitness.

Accessibility means your studio should be conveniently located for your target demographic. Use personas of your potential clients to find an accessible location. For instance, if you're targeting working professionals, a studio near office complexes or business parks would be strategic.

Visibility pertains to your studio's exposure. Choose a location prominently visible from main roads or commonly trafficked areas. Your studio itself can serve as an advertisement if placed correctly!

Community refers to the neighborhood demographics. Research surrounding areas for potential clients who might be inclined to yoga. Check for existing wellness establishments - gyms, organic cafes, health stores - these suggest that the community is health-conscious and open to yoga.

6.2. Selecting A Site

After determining the right neighborhood, begin your hunt for the perfect site. Keep in mind: Size, Sound, and Safety.

The Size of your studio will determine the number of students per class, impacting revenue. According to Yoga Alliance Standards, allow at least 20 square feet per student. Don't forget spaces for reception, changing rooms, and relaxation areas.

Sound plays a significant role in creating tranquility. Choose a site away from noisy areas, or invest in soundproofing. Ambient sounds can be beneficial if they align with the yoga experience, like a site near a garden for chirping birds.

Safety is paramount — both in terms of the structure and neighborhood security. Make sure the site passes all safety regulations. A secure neighborhood leads to a consistent client-flow, even for late-night or early-morning classes.

6.3. Designing Your Studio

At the heart of your yoga studio is its design — a physical manifestation of your vision. A carefully designed studio can enhance the yoga experience and keep students returning.

The Reception: It should exude warmth, making visitors feel welcome. Keep the space open, organized, and naturally lit, using warm colors and soft textures. Place schedules, registration desks, and merchandise, neatly. Add indoor plants for freshness.

The Practice Room: The most sacred space, should be serene, spacious, and minimal. Opt for neutral or earth tones. Provide ample space between mats, ensuring personal comfort. Soundproof the room, utilize diffused lighting and if possible, incorporate natural elements like a water feature.

Changing Rooms: Design for comfort and convenience. Provide lockers, multiple shower cubicles, and bathroom stalls. Install full-length mirrors and a vanity space. Maintaining sound hygiene is crucial.

Relaxation Spaces: They provide a spot to unwind pre/post classes. Comfy chairs, a small library, or even a tea corner enhances community vibes.

6.4. Layout Planning

A well-planned layout optimizes space, encourages fluid movement, and subtly communicates operational procedures to clients — from registration, changing, practicing, to relaxation.

Pay attention to the 'Flow of Movement'. Keep the registration desk in front, guiding students to changing rooms then the practice area. Post-practice, guide them through the relaxation space towards the exit. Place signage effectively.

Think about 'Space Maximization'. Multi-purpose furniture, efficient storage, vertical shelves all help optimize your studio's space.

Consider 'Aesthetic Accents'. A well-placed Buddha statue or a calming wall art can bring in tremendous character to your studio, making it memorable.

Never underestimated the power of 'Natural Elements'. Wherever possible, integrate natural light, greenery, or water bodies.

6.5. Adapting Design Over Time

Your studio should evolve with your business. Keep observing how space is used. Identify congested areas or underutilized corners. Gather feedback from students about their comfort. Be open to making phased changes to your layout or design. Regular refurbishment keeps your studio vibrant and fresh.

Remember, your yoga studio is more than just a business; it's a platform to transform lives through the power of yoga. Make sure it radiates positive energy, tranquility, and the promise of growth — bearing the comforting aura of a spiritual retreat right in the heart of a bustling city. With thoughtful location selection and mindful design, you are all set to create a yoga studio that you and your students will love. Happy Yoga-preneurship!

Chapter 7. Recruiting and Managing Your Yoga Team

Building a team is not only about hiring people who can execute yoga poses perfectly or have a deep understanding of yoga traditions. A great team involves like-minded individuals who align with your vision, mission, and culture.

7.1. Identifying Your Needs

Your first step towards recruiting your yoga team involves understanding your studio's needs. Ask yourself what kind of community you want to build and how your team will help build that. For example, if you want to focus on therapeutic yoga, you'll need teachers who specialize in this area.

Determine whether you need part-time or full-time instructors. Identify the style of yoga that you wish to offer - this could be ashtanga, yin, hatha, vinyasa, or even a blend of different styles. You may even need non-teaching staff such as administrative professionals, cleaners, and marketing personnel who are crucial for the successful operation of your studio.

7.2. Hiring Yoga Instructors

Recruiting a top-notch team begins with defining the perfect job description. Clearly spell out what you expect from your instructors in terms of skills, qualifications, experience, and style of teaching. Promote your job advertisements via your studio's website, social media platforms, and other specialised health and wellness job forums for maximum exposure.

This is an arena where you must not hesitate to be picky. Choosing the right yoga instructor is just as crucial as your business location or the services you offer.

7.3. Managing Your Team

Once you've gathered your team, your focus should then shift to management. Good leadership not only ensures the smooth operation of your studio but also plays a significant role in retaining your team.

Remember, your team is the heart and soul of your yoga studio. Treat them well, and they will, in turn, treat your clients well. Maintain an open line of communication with them. Acknowledge their good work and provide constructive feedback for improvement.

7.4. Staff Training

Conduct regular training and development programs to ensure that your instructors keep up with the latest practices in the field of yoga. Encourage them to attend yoga seminars and workshops. You may want to consider investing in their advanced training.

7.5. Setting Up Schedules

Setting up a schedule that works for everyone could be a bit of a challenge, especially if your team consists of part-time workers or those who juggle other commitments. To meet this challenge, use scheduling software. It simplifies the process of managing and organizing employee schedules. Ensure that your studio has appropriate coverage at all times.

7.6. Conflict Resolution

Conflicts may emerge due to personality clashes, miscommunication, or other issues. It's essential to address these conflicts promptly before they escalate. Create a peaceful but clear procedure to handle conflict resolution. Be fair, objective, and open-minded.

7.7. Employee Retention

Retention is crucial for building a successful yoga business. Invest in your staff. Consider offering perks like free yoga sessions, discounted training, or even incentives tied to the performance of the business.

By instilling a sense of belonging, appreciation, and mutual respect, you create an environment where your instructors want to stay and grow.

7.8. Legal Considerations

Ensure all legal aspects are in place. Your instructors should be correctly classified as either independent contractors or employees. Consult with an attorney to understand the legal implications of either categorization. Always ensure you comply with state and local employment laws.

Remember, your yoga team is not just a workforce; they are the pillars of your yoga community. By finding the right people, training them well, treating them with respect, and managing them effectively, you assure the success and longevity of your yoga studio.

Chapter 8. Building a Welcoming Studio Culture

Creating a warm and welcoming culture in your yoga studio could very well be the difference between a successful venture and a failed experiment. This chapter focuses on the elements to consider when building a culture that attracts and retains yoga enthusiasts.

8.1. The Importance of an Embracing Culture

A welcoming studio culture goes beyond aesthetics - it's about creating an environment where every student feels valued and included, regardless of their yoga proficiency level. A nurturing, engaged, inclusive, and community-focused culture can foster a high degree of student loyalty and commitment.

Hence, it is indispensable to invest the necessary energy, time, and resources into building a strong, welcoming, and enchanted studio culture that becomes the cornerstone of your yoga business. The effect of your exceptional yoga culture will reverberate beyond your walls, attracting potential clients and eliciting positive word-of-mouth referrals.

8.2. Creating an Authentic Mission and Vision

Everything begins with a clear purpose. Identify your mission statement - the guiding principle behind your studio's existence. It should resonate with your target audience and reflect your core beliefs about yoga and wellness.

Similarly, your vision statement should paint a picture of what you want your yoga studio to achieve. It could be enriching lives through yoga or fostering a community of mindfulness, for instance.

When your mission and vision are clearly articulated and conveyed, they will serve as the foundational pillar of your studio culture, attracting people who resonate with your brand identity.

8.3. Prioritizing Community Connections

Building a strong and interconnected community is crucial in creating a nurturing yoga studio culture. Emphasize human connections and give your attendees a chance to interact – before, during, and after the classes. Encourage local collaborations, host community events or wellness workshops, and become a part of local festivals and markets. By doing so, your studio becomes a hub for community interaction.

8.4. Ensuring Diversity and Inclusivity

Encourage folks of all ages, genders, races, and backgrounds to join your studio by offering classes at varying skill levels and different yoga styles. Aim for a diverse and inclusive teacher pool who can cater to, and connect with, this wide demographic.

Moreover, incorporate inclusivity in your communication - both offline and online. Make efforts to ensure your content, images, and marketing materials communicate the message that "everyone is welcome."

8.5. Building a Team that Reflects Your Culture

Hiring the right teachers and staff members who align with your studio's culture is pivotal. They are the face of your brand and directly influence the culture of your yoga studio. Motivate staff with regular trainings, fostering a team that's empathetic, respectful, and knowledgeable. Transparent communication about your expectations regarding culture can help them stay aligned with your vision.

8.6. Offering Superior Customer Service

Exceptional customer service is essential to your studio's reputation. Respond to inquiries promptly, handle issues with patience and tact, and create a consistent positive experience for your clients. The little things matter - a friendly greeting, remembering names, or offering a cup of herbal tea can go a long way.

8.7. Seeking Regular Feedback

Feedback mechanisms are great for keeping a pulse on your studio culture. Provide opportunities for students and staff to share suggestions and concerns. Regularly using surveys or suggestion boxes can help you understand their needs and preferences, allowing you to continue tweaking and enhancing your culture.

8.8. Encouraging Personal Growth

Promote personal growth among your students and staff alike. Encourage self-exploration and discovery, be it through meditation workshops, mindfulness sessions, or yoga retreats. This way, your studio becomes more than just a place to practice yoga; it's a sanctuary of growth and self-discovery.

In conclusion, building a welcoming yoga studio culture is an ongoing process and one that requires dedication, passion, and a deep understanding of your target audience. However, the rewards - a loyal customer base, active word-of-mouth marketing, and a thriving community - make these efforts well worth it.

Chapter 9. Marketing Magic: Promote, Advertise, and Sustain

Success is not just a function of a stellar product or service, but also expert promotion, advertising, and sustainability mechanisms. For any entrepreneur, mastering marketing magic is instrumental.

9.1. Understanding the Market

Understanding the market is the first step toward successful marketing. Familiarize yourself with the demographics, preferred styles of yoga, pricing strategies of competing studios, and lifestyle factors influencing your potential customers. Recognize that your clientele will likely consist of a wide spectrum of individuals, including early risers, lunch break yogis, evening practitioners, beginners, seasoned yogis, and even youth classes.

Use surveys or publicly available data to gather detailed demographic information. Once armed with this data, aim to provide services that align with those specific needs.

9.2. Choosing the Right Message

Messaging is crucial when marketing given that it creates connections with potential customers. It should resonate with your target audience emotionally and communicate the unique value of practicing yoga at your studio. What set your studio apart? Is it the serene setting, the top-notch instructors, or the variety of classes you offer?

When crafting your messaging, be consistent and true to your brand.

Strive to inspire, motivate, and connect on a personal, emotional level.

9.3. Traditional Marketing Strategies

Traditional marketing methods can still prove useful, even in our digital age. This could include advertisements in local newspapers, radio stations, billboards, or flyers distributed within the community. Networking can also play a fundamental role in traditional marketing tactics. Form partnerships with local businesses and offer them corporate wellness packages; this will not only create relationships but also offer advertising through word-of-mouth.

9.4. Digital Marketing Strategies

In today's digital landscape, effective online marketing is vital. Harness the power of social media to build an online persona that accurately represents your brand. Platforms such as Facebook, Instagram, and Twitter can be useful in promoting your studio and engaging with potential and current clients. Ensure that your content is engaging, consistent, and speaks to your target audience.

SEO (Search Engine Optimization) is another digital marketing strategy that can dramatically increase your studio's visibility online. By optimizing your website's content to appear in the top search results, you attract more organic traffic, and by extension, more potential clients.

9.5. Utilizing Reviews and Testimonials

Customer testimonials are essentially positive votes for your yoga studio. Request for reviews from your satisfied clients and show them on your website or share them on social media channels. They provide social proof, and prospective members are more likely to trust reviews from actual clients.

9.6. Hosting Events and Workshops

Hosting events and workshops are another great way to draw people to your yoga studio. They are excellent promotional tools as they allow people to experience your services firsthand. Open houses, free trial classes, community events, and workshops on specific yoga styles or wellness topics can all generate excitement and interest in your studio.

9.7. Retaining Members

While attracting new customers is essential, retaining existing members is even more crucial for sustainable growth. Offer membership benefits, additional services like spa or wellness centers, or yoga merchandise to boost retention. Furthermore, ensure your pricing policies are transparent, fair, and offer value to your members.

9.8. Measuring Marketing Success

Once you have implemented your marketing strategies, it's crucial to track their effectiveness. Some metrics to consider include: customer acquisition cost, customer lifetime value, member retention rate, and online engagement rates. Tracking these metrics helps identify what's working and areas for improvement in your marketing efforts.

Mastering the art of marketing your yoga studio is not an overnight process. It requires continuous learning, assessment, and adaptation.

Follow these steps to create a dynamic marketing strategy that attracts, retains, and delights your members, ensuring the sustainability and success of your yoga studio. Make way for prosperity and tranquility as you embark on this rewarding entrepreneurial journey into the world of yoga.

Chapter 10. Expanding Horizons: Classes, Workshops, and Special Events

Starting your yoga studio essentially involves designing a space where community and self-realization meet, a place that enables individuals to connect with their inner selves and thrive in their yoga practices. The key to a flourishing yoga studio doesn't stop at the door of a simple yoga class; your studio's blueprint must encompass diverse classes, workshops, and special events. Let's delve into the details of diversifying your yoga offerings and creating a thriving, dynamic yoga community.

10.1. Expanding your Class Offerings

Think beyond basic yoga classes. Once you establish a recurring clientele, consider introducing a variety of yoga styles to offer something for everyone. From Vinyasa to Ashtanga, Yin to Restorative, different styles cater to different needs and preferences.

Some other popular yoga styles to consider are: * Power yoga: Ideal for those seeking a vigorous workout. * Bikram yoga: Hot yoga conducted in high-temperature rooms. * Kundalini yoga: Focusing on consciousness and self-awareness through motion and meditation. * Iyengar yoga: Emphasis on alignment, sequence, and timing. * Hatha yoga: A slow-paced class focusing on breathing techniques and core yoga poses.

Offering multi-level classes is also beneficial to tend to yoga practitioners of different experience levels. These could range from beginner classes to intermediate and advanced levels, with proper guidance and attention given to beginners transitioning into intermediate stages and so forth.

10.2. Running Regular Workshops

Once your audience grows and you've nurtured a solid community of yoga students, hosting workshops can be a game-changer. Workshops deepen the knowledge and practice of yoga, either by focusing on a specific style, practice (like inversions or arm balances), or integrating other holistic practices such as Ayurveda, meditation, or yoga philosophy.

You can consider workshops like: * Yoga Anatomy: This helps students understand the biomechanics of yoga poses. * Yoga for Wellness: This could cover topics like stress management, nutrition, or yoga for mental health. * Chakra Balancing Workshop: Teach about energy balancing and techniques for achieving wellness. * Partner Yoga or Acroyoga workshops: Offer something fun and build connections within your yoga community.

Instructors for workshops could include in-house teachers or visiting experts. Make sure that these workshops offer value to your students beyond their regular classes and leave them craving for more insights.

10.3. Organizing Special Events

Special events are a brilliant way to create a community outside of regular classes and workshops. These can be anything from a sunrise beach yoga session, yoga retreats in nature, to charity yoga classes, wellness festivals or events celebrating International Yoga Day.

Remember that events should be inclusive, welcoming everyone from your regular students to beginners, and even those who have never stepped on a yoga mat. This way, you not only provide an intriguing and fun event for your existing members but also attract potential new members to your studio.

10.4. Collaborating with other Wellness Practices

A holistic approach to wellness is becoming increasingly popular. Consider partnering with nutritional coaches, psychologists, mindfulness experts, or physiotherapists to provide holistic wellness programs. This could range from diet plan guidance to stress management to rehabilitation aid.

10.5. Implementing a Tiered Pricing System

Your pricing needs to align with your offerings. Implementing a tiered pricing system can ensure that you get adequate returns on the quality services you provide. You can offer class packages, early-bird discounts for workshops and special events, or VIP memberships for regular clients.

In conclusion, expanding your offerings is one of the most enriching steps you could take, not only for your yoga studio but also for your yoga community. The idea is to provide a space that meets the needs of varying individuals, making yoga accessible and enjoyable for everyone. Welcoming people into a space where they feel comfortable exploring their practice ensures they develop loyalty to your studio. Your yoga studio can truly become a hub of well-being, a community of vibrant, joyful, and peaceful people, and ultimately, a flourishing yoga business. Remember, your success will come 'one peaceful inhale and successful exhale at a time'.

Chapter 11. Finding Your Balance: Growth, Profitability, and Peace

Starting your yoga business requires not only a deep-seated passion for yoga, but a keen eye for balancing growth, profitability, and peace. This chapter aims to guide you through these crucial components of your journey towards building a successful yoga enterprise.

11.1. Setting a Vision for Your Business

To find balance, you must first dream. Where do you want your business to be in one year? What about in five years? Setting a vision for your yoga studio will provide a guiding light as you navigate through the complex world of growth and profitability. It also gives you a benchmark for success and helps in crafting your business plan, setting your marketing strategy, and making tactical and financial decisions.

Take a moment to draw on your personal goals and aspirations for your yoga studio. Consider your desired location, the diversity of classes you offer, the number of employees, students and the atmosphere you would like to create. This vision will serve as your compass, always pointing you in the direction of your dream yoga studio.

11.2. Embracing Growth Mindset

The next step in this equilibrium-seeking journey is fostering a growth mindset. You must cultivate an open mind, ready to embrace changes and adapt to the dynamic nature of business.

Understanding your demographic, their needs and preferences, and the trends in the yoga industry will enable you to consistently fine-tune your service offerings and studio environment. Whether it's considering new yoga styles, implementing innovative teaching methods, or providing attractive packages, incorporating growth factors will ensure the longevity and prosperity of your studio.

11.3. Profitability - The Financial Balance

A successful yoga business relies on its financial health. Profitability doesn't only mean having a positive net income at the end of the year; it entails sustaining your business during lean periods and investing back into it to foster growth.

Determine your breakeven point - how many classes you need to hold per week, how many students per class, and the price per class. Be cognizant of your overhead costs such as rent, salaries, utilities, and taxes. Conducting a regular financial review will help you fill gaps, cut unnecessary costs, and improve the overall financial health of your business.

11.4. Pricing Strategy

Your pricing strategy plays a vital role in determining your profitability. Your class prices should cover your costs while attracting and retaining your preferred clientele. Research the market, understand what similar studios are charging, and determine what your prospective students are willing to pay.

Keep in mind the value your classes offer. If your studio provides a unique experience, top-notch instructors, or specialized classes, you could justify higher prices. Meanwhile, offering discounts or tiered memberships can also be a strategic way to grow your customer base and increase session frequency.

11.5. Harnessing Peace

Your yoga studio isn't simply a business; it's your sanctuary. Amid the logistics of growth, profit analysis, and business strategies, don't lose sight of your core: bringing peace. Heed your ethos of creating spaces where people can seek tranquility and empowerment through yoga. This balance between your passion and the operational demands of your business is central to your success.

11.6. Mindful Marketing

Marketing strategies can boost customer acquisition and retention. From social media and email campaigns to webinars and community events, each marketing avenue should align with your vision and the peaceful aura you wish to promulgate.

Embrace mindful marketing, an approach that focuses on understanding your audience's needs and delivering content in a conscious, purposeful manner. It requires you to be genuine and communicative, building deep connections with your community. This will not only help grow your customer base but also foster a loyalty that extends beyond classes and packages.

11.7. Building a Resilient Team

No yoga business is complete without its team. You must carefully select instructors and staff who resonate with your vision. Invest in them, train them, and ensure they feel valued. A resilient team is key to managing the ebb and flow of business. They reflect your business's ethos and contribute to building an environment where your students feel comfortable and connected.

11.8. Conclusion

Finding the balance between growth, profitability, and peace might seem like a challenging tightrope walk. It's a dynamic quest that requires constant awareness and adjustment. But armed with a clear vision, a growth mindset, financial acumen, mindful marketing, strategic pricing, and a resilient team, you will surely master the art of 'Yoga-preneurship.' Embrace this journey of creating a successful yoga studio that benefits not only the body and mind, but also the wallet.